Alkaline Diet: The Scientifically Proven Way to Lose Weight and Fight Against Chronic Disease

I0146061

By Jason Michaels

that are mentioned are done without written consent and can in no way be considered an endorsement from the trademark holder.

Medical Disclaimer
This book is not intended as a substitute for the medical advice of physicians. The reader should regularly consult a physician in matters relating to his/her health and particularly with respect to any symptoms that may require diagnosis or medical attention.

Please consult your physician before starting any diet or exercise program.

Any recommendations given in this book are not a substitute for medical advice.

Table of Contents

Introduction

Congratulations on downloading this book, and thank you for doing so.

The following chapters will discuss all about the alkaline diet and how it can help improve your health. We'll be clearing up all the misconceptions and setting the record straight on how the life-extending diet can dramatically improve your health.

A lot of people consume the wrong types of food which causes them diseases, chronic conditions, and even premature aging.

If you learn about the benefits of an alkaline diet, you will be able to make adjustments to your eating habits and lifestyle to lead a healthier and more fulfilling life.

An alkaline diet does your body a lot of good. It helps to prevent diseases such as cancer and also helps to manage chronic conditions like hypertension. We'll be discussing which foods are alkaline (there's a lot of confusion about which are, and which aren't), and precisely why alkaline foods are better than acidic foods.

Thanks again for choosing this book! Every effort was made to ensure it is full of as much useful information as possible. I hope you enjoy reading and get the maximum possible benefits out of it.

Jason Michaels

Chapter 1: An Introduction to the Alkaline Diet

What is the alkaline diet? The term alkaline diet refers to a group of diets that are closely related based on the fact that different food types can affect the body's pH balance.

The alkaline diet supports the consumption of green leafy vegetables, lots of fruits, nuts, salads, seeds and drinking alkaline water. The diet discourages the consumption of foods such as eggs, grains, cheese, and some meats. Other foods that negatively impact the body and cause acidity include dairy, burgers, sweets, cola, beer, chocolate, and chips.

To lead a healthy lifestyle, a person needs to ensure that at least 70% of their food is alkaline, and the acidic foods should be limited as much as possible.

The diet is very simple and provides a realistic approach to health. The human body functions best in an alkaline state. This is because it is designed to remain and operate best when in an alkaline state. The body does everything it can to remain in this state. The problem is that when we consume unhealthy, acidic foods, then our bodies become overwhelmed by acidity, and this can result in serious consequences. The situation is made worse when a person does not exercise, is stressed, and hardly gets sufficient sleep.

The Life-Extending, Disease-Fighting Alkaline Diet

While there are plenty of varied diets out there, none is more effective for staving off disease and longevity that the alkaline diet. It has been established that such a diet can help balance your body's pH levels. This will result in a significant reduction in mortality and morbidity of different chronic illnesses such as diabetes, arthritis, hypertension, low bone density, and Vitamin D deficiency.

This is according to a review published in 2012 in the *American Journal of Environmental Health*. There have been numerous claims about the alkaline diet not just preventing but also helping rid the body of conditions such as cancer.

How Do Alkaline Diets Work? It is an established fact, according to research, that a diet rich in plant-based unprocessed proteins, fruits, leafy vegetables, and essential minerals causes the urine's pH to lower, and this helps balance mineral levels and also provides protection to the cells within the body.

The pH level of the body is mainly determined by the mineral content of the foods a person consumes. Just like temperature, pH levels are regulated by the body to keep them as close to normal levels as possible. The average pH of a healthy person is slightly over 7, about

7.4, which is slightly alkaline. All life forms and living organisms exist simply because their bodies maintain appropriate pH levels. It is believed that no disease can affect a pH-Balanced body. According to scientists, the human body requires a strictly controlled pH level that ranges between 7.35 and 7.45, depending on some factors such as last time a person used the bathroom; what they ate; their diet; and the time of day.When a person consumes too much of the wrong food types and develops an electrolyte imbalance, he or she is likely to suffer from acidosis.

What Is Acidosis? This is a situation where the body contains too much acid that the lungs and kidneys cannot maintain the required pH balance. A lot of the processes within the body often result in acidity. The lungs and kidneys can compensate for minor pH changes. This is because the acidity in the body is always a result of either respiration or metabolism.

Any pH level that is lower than 7.35 is considered acidic. Any pH level above 7.45 is alkaline. While the difference may seem small, the significance of each is huge.

The History of the Alkaline Diet

In recent years, the alkaline diet has become increasingly popular. However, the concept of an alkaline diet had been acknowledged as early as the 1920s. Scientists have studied the role of diet and its influence on urine acidity for many years.

According to nutrition scientists of the early 20th century, food contains both negatively and positively charged particles. Diets that are rich in sulfate, phosphate, and chloride were presumed to be acidic while those that contain calcium, potassium, and magnesium were presumed to be alkaline forming.

Over the years, scientists developed different theories of alkalinity and acidity. The pH scale, which was invented in 1909, assisted scientists to determine the acidity and alkaline nature of foods. pH stands for the potential for hydrogen, and it is a measure of the number of hydrogen ions in a given volume of fluid.

New York doctor William H. Hay first spoke about the benefits of an alkaline diet. He put down his thoughts in some books that include *Weight Control* and *Health Via Food*. The diet has made a resurgence starting in 2003 after the release of another publication, *The pH Miracle*. The media has helped to mainstream the alkaline diet and increase its popularity around the world.

Dr. Sebi and T. Colin Campbell

Dr. Sebi

Dr. Sebi was a Honduran health and wellness expert whose extensive work in the field of natural health resulted in the creation of a specialized diet. He believed that there are generally six major food groups. These are raw, hybrid, dead, live, drugs, and genetically modified. When he modified a diet based on these major food groups, he eliminated all food groups and only stuck with raw and live. He encouraged people to consume meals that are as close to raw vegan as possible. Many enthusiasts often refer to a list of foods that consist of what he referred to as the best of the alkaline diet. This is known as the Dr. Sebi Product List and is very popular with health enthusiasts around the world.

Thomas Colin Campbell, PhD

T Colin Campbell is an American biochemist who has performed extensive research in nutrition research and education. His work has focused closely on the relationship between disease and diet and in particular, cancer. The China Project, one of his numerous projects, is still considered one of the most comprehensive research studies of nutrition and health ever conducted.

Campbell is well known for advocating for whole foods, and low-fat, plant-based diets. Apart from authoring more than 3 books and over 300 research papers, he remains one of the most popular health and nutrition authors after his book, *The China Study*, became a best-seller in the nutrition genre.

PH Levels and the Human Body

The pH of any substance is essentially a measure of how acidic or alkaline it is. The human body regulates pH levels to keep it in great condition. There are plenty of organs that play a huge role in this field. Other factors that affect the body's pH levels include medications, diet, and exercise.

A pH measure of 7.0 is largely considered neutral. Anything above this is alkaline while any number below is acidic. PH measures hydrogen ions in the body. Water is neutral and has a pH level of 7.0. The human blood maintains a pH level of about 7.4 which makes it slightly alkaline.

Why is pH Important?

A lot of the time, people consume foods that are very acidic. When the body becomes acidic, it has to reach out to its alkaline reserves to neutralize the acidity. Magnesium, calcium, and potassium are drawn from the bones and tissues to raise the body's pH levels.

Plenty of the ailments that are faced by an ordinary person are as a result of acidity within the body. Take the case where the blood is too acidic. The body will line the arteries with fat to prevent them from getting corroded. This, in turn, raises the risk of cardiovascular conditions.

Also, when the body has to get alkaline reserves from the bones, then the risk of conditions such as osteoporosis as well as loss of bone density are all matters of great concern. Bacteria are known to thrive in acidic bodies. They are responsible for a myriad of problems within the body including anxiety, depression, and other cognitive and psychological disorders. It is, therefore, crucial to regularly check the body's pH levels and to alkalize the body.

The Alkaline Diet vs. Paleo Diet

The Paleo diet is often referred to as caveman's diet. This is because its emphasis is on adopting the eating lifestyles of our early ancestors. The diet focuses on consuming foods such as nuts, eggs, seafood, vegetables, fruits, lean meat, fermented foods, healthy fats, and seeds.

On the other hand, the alkaline diet compromises 20% acidic foods and 80% alkaline foods. This diet emphasizes the right kinds of nuts, vegetables, and seeds. Healthy fats and sugary fruits are not allowed. It also requires one to check their pH levels regularly. It involves testing urine for acidity levels.

The Paleo diet allows consumption of lean meat and fruits while the alkaline diet forbids most of these as they are not alkaline. The alkaline diet also forbids dairy, grains, seafood, starches, fermented foods, and dried foods. Also, regular exercise and plenty of sleep are essential.

Myths about the Alkaline Diet

1. It is too difficult to stick with. This is not true because there are plenty of people who diligently follow this diet and related lifestyles.

2. Alkaline diet meals are boring. There are plenty of delicious alkaline meals
Other myths include the fact that followers of the alkaline lifestyle cannot enjoy treats anymore, that they will not get sufficient dairy, potassium, calcium, and proteins. Another myth claims that the alkaline diet is only for weight loss purposes.

Do You Have to be Vegan?

Generally, a lot of people assume that an alkaline diet is akin to a vegan diet. An alkaline diet is mostly vegan but not entirely. In fact, plenty of people often ask if they have to give up their meats to practice the alkaline diet.

The alkaline food chart indicates that fish and goat's cheese, for instance, as only moderately acidic. This means they can be consumed together with highly alkaline foods. The aim is often to consume a meal that is 70 – 80% alkaline and 20 – 30% acidic. Another important aspect to keep in mind is to consume grass-fed beef, bacon from properly raised pigs, and butter from pasture-raised cattle.

One of the bigger misconceptions is whether you need to be vegan or not to get the maximum benefits. Although the alkaline diet generally discourages the consumption of refined sugars and processed foods. It calls for consumption of more greens and plenty of veggies. However, it should be noted that animal fat and protein will not necessarily increase acidity in the body. A vegan diet is, therefore, only an option but is not a requirement; neither is it necessary for anyone considering the alkaline diet. Once again, this is a big myth in the alkaline community - you do NOT have to be vegan to get all the benefits on an alkaline diet.

Chapter 2: Human Diet Changes Over the Past 100 Years - And How Our Health Has Worsened

It is a fact that the human diet has changed more in the past one hundred years than in the previous 4 million years. Our eating habits have changed immensely. We can hardly compare our diets today with those of our grandparents. Some experts think we should revert to a Stone Age menu. Our attitudes towards diet have altered the way we shop, what we buy, cook, and how we dine.

About a hundred years ago, our grandparents and great-grandparents stuck to strict meal times. Breakfast was probably at 7.00 am, lunch at 12.00 noon, and dinner at 5.00 pm. Such strict routines adhered to about a hundred years ago accustomed the body to know when to expect nutrition. The disciplined mealtimes also helped keep waists rather trim, and food wastage was unheard of.

The modern lifestyle has changed a lot, and people do not adhere to strict mealtimes anymore. People also consume more than three meals each day. Some skip breakfast; others have mid-morning snacks; many others enjoy numerous cups of coffee throughout the day.

Healthier Foods

A century ago, most of the food consumed was freshly harvested from the farms or bought at the market. Common foods back then included fresh vegetables, eggs, beef, whole milk, pork, fruits, fish, and even the good, healthy fats. Back then, there were hardly any reported cases of heart disease, high blood pressure, and so on.

However, with increased populations and expansion of cities, people started to abandon healthy lifestyles and opted for unhealthy choices. For instance, animal fat was abandoned as it was believed to be unhealthy. Over the years, they moved to refined carbohydrates, desserts, pasta, grains, bread, and omega-6 fatty acids.

Industrialization of Food Is Hurting Our Bodies

Factory-farmed foods are now more common than ever. About 10 billion farm animals, excluding fish and marine organisms, will be raised in commercial farms this year alone. A hundred years ago, such a huge industry was actually inconceivable. Most families lived in a rural or a small town setting where fresh produce was readily available.

The rest who lived in large towns and cities had dairy products such as milk delivered to them fresh from the farm. Other products such as eggs and meat were fresh and readily available at the local butchery. Our great-grandparents and grandparents ate these foods in plenty and hardly fell sick. This is because they consumed healthy animal products, those raised outdoors, on grass, and with plenty of human love.

Today, animals kept for produce are fed all sorts of artificial feeds including genetically modified feed, food with growth hormones, and even antibiotics. More and more animals are now raised in factories and never eat any natural food. Instead, they consume unnatural, manufactured food loaded with drugs and a myriad of chemicals. These have a huge impact on the humans that consume them.

Fruits and vegetables conventionally grown contain fewer minerals and vitamins today than they did about a century or so ago. The reason can be attributed to the widespread use of chemical fertilizers and pesticides. These tend to disrupt the quality of the soil and affect the nutrients. Runoff water from the farms contains chemical fertilizers and other pollutants. This poisoned water ends up in our rivers and lakes and affects the birds, fish, and other species within the same ecosystem.

Processed Foods

Many decades ago, food was a huge part of the culture. However, there was no junk food back then. All meals were healthy, fresh, and natural. Real food was highly valued. However, things began to change in the 1950s. It was then that the idea of fast foods and shortcuts started. The idea was to prepare food faster but keep it healthy and balanced.

In America alone, 80% of the processed foods consumed contain genetically modified ingredients. The fast foods consumed now hardly resemble those consumed in the 1950s and did not exist 100 years ago. Processed foods contain huge amounts of artificial colors, preservatives, sweeteners, and flavors, and are packaged in plastic. This makes fast foods consumed today absolutely unhealthy and a risk to human health.

Processed foods constitute some of the major reasons why people around the world are becoming obese and suffering chronic conditions like cancer, high blood pressure, diabetes, and many more.

As a matter of necessity, most foods are processed in some way. For instance, cheese is produced from milk; peanuts are processed to produce peanut butter, and bread is baked after preparing the dough. However, mechanic processing of food is totally different from chemical processing.

The latter produces unhealthy and dangerous fast foods and junk foods like soda, candy, chips, cookies, and so on. These foods will not only make you fat and overweight; they will affect the quality of your life, make you age prematurely, and even make you sick.

Most processed foods contain sugars such as corn syrup. These sugars are very addictive and often deplete the body of essential nutrients. The nature of high- fructose corn syrup is such that it encourages continuous eating by affecting the regulating hormone, leptin. This is why people consume such high quantities of junk food. This definitely leads to obesity and other issues.

The preservatives used are often dangerous and harmful to human health. A lot of the junk foods on the shelves of department stores have a shelf life of 10 years or more. This is a great reason to worry because a lot of the preservatives used to stabilize fats are possible carcinogenic and can cause cancer.

Processed foods and junk foods have introduced a culture of mindless eating. People will nowadays spend hours sitting down watching TV or using a computer while all the time eating continuously. Such mindless consumption of junk food has a hugely negative impact on our overall health.

Coloring in foods, while approved for use by the authorities, is not good for the human body. Research has linked some food coloring to attention deficit disorder and attention deficit hyperactivity disorder in kids. Other types of food coloring such as caramel actually contain known carcinogens.

Artificial flavors are even worse because they are a blanket term and are not even named. This is different from food colors which are all known. Artificial flavors generally refer to hundreds of different chemical flavors that are created to imitate natural flavors. Nobody ever gets to know what's been added to any food that contains artificial flavors.

It is therefore advisable to avoid chemically processed foods,especially junk foods. Mechanically processed foods are okay as long as they are of high quality.

Naturally processed foods that contain no additives are okay for human consumption.

Diseases Caused by High Salt Intake and Processed Foods

High Salt Intake

We love salt in food because it makes it tasty and adds a nice flavor to it. Food without salt is bland and doesn't appeal to the taste buds. However, excessive consumption of salt can result in serious conditions. For a long time, scientists have associated high salt levels with high blood pressure and cardiovascular problems.

In most people, high salt consumption causes trouble for the kidneys. The kidneys are forced to overwork trying to eliminate excess sodium in the blood. The body also holds onto water in an attempt to dissolve and dilute the sodium. This results in increased blood volume and fluid within the cells. The heart is forced to work harder, and the blood vessels are strained. With time, this results in hypertension or high blood pressure. Other conditions likely to follow include heart attacks, strokes, and other cardiovascular conditions.

Excessive salt in the body can also result in heart failure. Also, the heart, aorta, and kidneys will be damaged due to overworking. Excessive salt is also bad for the bones. High blood pressure, which is closely associated with excessive amounts of salt in the diet, is the main cause of heart disease. 50% of all heart diseases and 67% of all strokes are as a result of high blood pressure.

Salt is present in high quantities in processed foods, and these are found in most homes and are consumed throughout the day. The recommended salt intake per person per day, according to the World Health Organization is five grams. High salt diets can result in multiple sclerosis, delayed puberty, enlarged muscle tissue, and damage to internal organs.

Processed Foods

Processed foods are unhealthy because of the chemical processes they are put through and the numerous additives such as preservatives and artificial colors they contain. They are huge contributors to illnesses and obesity all over the world.

Often people misunderstand what the term "processed foods" means. Food can be chemically or mechanically processed. Mechanically processed foods such as ground beef or orange juice are okay. The problem is with the chemically processed foods. These are produced using artificial substances and refined ingredients. Such foods are bad for your health.

Processed foods contain large amounts of sugars such as corn syrup. It contains no calories but is high in energy. This can result in problems such as increased levels of bad cholesterol, high triglycerides, and insulin resistance. The sugar in highly processed foods can cause plenty of challenges to our health. For instance, it devastatingly affects metabolism.

A lot of people do not add sugar to their coffee or cereal. They are getting it from the processed foods they eat and sugary drinks they take. Beverages and processed foods contain massive amounts of sugar. Sugar is extremely unhealthy and has serious consequences for the health of consumers.

Processed foods contain plenty of artificial ingredients. A lot of the time, consumers are not able to understand the contents of packaged and processed foods that they buy. The reason is that most of the ingredients are actually not food but chemicals added for different purposes. Processed foods such as potato chips and candy are highly addictive.

The sugars activate sections of the brain that are also affected by hard drugs such as cocaine. It is a fact that junk food affects the biochemistry of the brain, and this can lead to addiction and loss of control over eating habits.

Highly processed foods contain almost no nutrients. They also contain simple carbohydrates which are highly refined and add no value to the body. They instead lead to spikes in blood sugar as well as an increase in insulin levels. This will in return have bad effects on your health. A lack of essential nutrients can also result in numerous other illnesses. Refined foods also lack fiber which is essential for good health.

Chapter 3: The Negative Effects of Acidosis

Electrolyte Imbalances

The term electrolyte imbalance refers to an abnormality in the body of the concentration of electrolytes. Electrolytes are chemicals such as potassium, sodium, magnesium, and others. They are the tiniest of all chemicals that are essential for proper functioning within the cells.

Electrolytes help to regulate neurological and heart function and also help to maintain homeostasis in the body. However, electrolyte imbalance can occur at any time due to some reasons. Excess elimination or reduced intake of electrolytes, excessive ingestion, and reduced elimination of an electrolyte are all reasons why imbalances may occur. Imbalance mostly occurs when the levels of potassium, calcium, sodium, or magnesium become abnormally low.

Electrolytes are extremely useful to the body. They enable cells such as muscle, heart, and nerve, to carry and transmit electrical signals. Kidneys are the organs that ensure there is no electrolyte imbalance in the body.

What is Acidosis?

This is a medical condition where the balance of acid and alkaline in blood plasma is affected such that there is excess acidity in the blood. Such blood will have a pH of 7.35 or below. Therefore, when the blood is acidic, then acidosis has occurred.

The body normally regulates the acidity of the blood. However, when it lasts for a long time, then it will weaken the body's immunity as all the internal systems will be weakened. This will make the body prone to diseases and illnesses. A healthy body generally protects against diseases, but in a weakened state, it is not able to function adequately. Excess acidity in the blood has to be neutralized in good time. However, the body may have to reach into its alkaline reserves to do this, and this leaves the body vulnerable to attacks.

Two Forms of Acidosis

There are generally two types of acidosis. There is respiratory acidosis that occurs when the body retains too much carbon dioxide, and then there is metabolic acidosis. This is often as a result when there is too much acid in the body. According to health professionals, acidosis occurs mostly due to conditions such as kidney or liver disease, chronic diarrhea, diabetes, and even respiratory diseases. Severe forms of acidosis are considered emergency cases because of their life-threatening nature.

The body is often fighting against viruses, bacteria, yeast, molds, and even fungi. This regular battling against pathogens tends to strengthen the immune system. Regular use of antibiotics tends to weaken the system, making the body vulnerable to germ attacks and diseases.

Acidosis and Ageing

According to modern science, acidosis is probably one of the main causes of premature aging. Most of the content of the food we eat consists of hydrogen, carbon, oxygen, and nitrogen. Only about 1% is minerals. When these products are digested, they release waste that is highly acidic. This waste usually exits the body via the kidneys and sweat. However, the acid that is not eliminated clogs the cells and circulates the body.

The residual acid that remains in the body deprives cells of oxygen and nutrients. Such cells and blood vessels become clogged, and this results in premature aging as well as serious health conditions. This is the main reason why people age.

Why Is Acidosis Bad for Your Health?

An acidic body is an unhealthy body because the human is designed to function optimally at slight alkaline levels. Acidosis simply implies there is too much acid in the body, and it will result in serious illnesses, if not checked.

Acidosis will initially cause an upset stomach. This will cause symptoms such as vomiting and nausea as well as decreased appetite. These symptoms are likely to persist and even get worse if the situation is not attended to.

Acidosis is likely to cause fatigue, headaches, and breathing difficulties. Vital organs will be starved of essential nutrients and oxygen. This makes the muscles feel weak, and fatigue will set in. It becomes difficult to focus on work or perform regular activities.

Abnormally high levels of acid in the blood can cause difficulty when breathing. This can lead to headaches, dizziness, and a fast heart rate. Other problems that can arise due to acidosis include coma, shock, and even death. Shock causes dizziness, pain in the chest region, sweating, and bluish skin color.

Chronically high acidosis levels are likely to result in severe health consequences such as loss of consciousness, organ failure, a coma, and eventual death. Seeking immediate relief from a health facility is important.

Acidosis Reduction for a Longer Life

If acidosis causes premature aging, then it follows that eliminating it would result in a longer, healthier life. One important and immediate solution is drinking alkaline water. Healthcare workers recommend consuming a low meat diet and plenty of vegetables. A vegan diet is largely recommended. Vegetables help to neutralize acidic waste.

Alkaline water is water that contains a higher percentage of oxygen than ordinary water. When alkaline water is consumed, it increases the amount of oxygen in the body which in turn neutralizes the acid in the cells.

Food Examples that Promote an Alkaline Body

Basically, food groups such as nuts, fruits, vegetables, and legumes will help to alkalize the body. Green leafy vegetables are the best as they contain high levels of important electrolytes like magnesium, potassium, and calcium. Also, plant-based proteins, all raw foods, and uncooked vegetables are said to be among the best sources of foods. Green drinks are great too. These are drinks made from grasses and green vegetables.

Chapter 4: How to Beat Hypertension

Blood Pressure

Blood pressure is a measure of the pressure exerted on blood vessel walls as the blood flows. The pressure is determined by the amount of resistance within the arteries as well as the amount of blood pumped by the heart.

Sometimes this pressure is high enough to cause health problems like kidney and heart disease. When the pressure is very high, the condition is known as high blood pressure. Basically, the narrower the blood vessels and the more blood that the heart pumps, the higher is the blood pressure.

The heart regularly pumps blood into blood vessels like arteries which then transport the blood throughout the body. Hypertension causes the heart to work much harder which results in complications such as kidney disease, stroke, heart conditions, and hardening of the arteries. Hypertension is, therefore, a very dangerous condition and should be adequately managed.

Normal Blood Pressure

Normal blood pressure is often quoted as 120 over 80. The initial number is referred to as systolic while the latter is diastolic. Figures above 180 over 120 are considered a crisis, and anyone with such levels should seek emergency medical attention. Blood pressure levels above what is considered normal should be lowered. Health practitioners can advise on ways to lower the blood pressure.

Causes of Hypertension

While the exact cause of hypertension remains unknown, certain factors are known as risk factors. They include obesity, too much salt in food, smoking, genetics, aging, chronic kidney disease, stress, and thyroid disorders. Secondary causes of high blood pressure or hypertension include congenital blood vessel defects, adrenal gland tumors, and obstructive sleep apnea. Other secondary causes are medications such as over-the-counter medications like painkillers, illegal drugs like amphetamines and cocaine, and chronic alcohol abuse.

Symptoms

High blood pressure never presents any symptoms. A person can suffer from hypertension for years without any symptoms at all. This condition develops over many years, and victims are often unaware of it. However, it continues to cause damage to internal organs such as kidneys, blood vessels, and the heart. If hypertension goes on for a long time, then it can result in serious health complications.

Checking your blood pressure on a regular basis is important. This way, any significant changes will be noted, and you can take action to control and manage the situation. It is also advisable to be on the lookout for the following risk factors:

Age: As we age, the risk of getting cancer also increases. From ages 40 to 50, high blood pressure becomes prevalent in men. However, women tend to develop the condition at age 65 and beyond.

Family history: People with a history of high blood pressure are more likely to suffer from this condition than others.

Race: Statistics indicate that hypertension is prevalent among dark-skinned communities such as African Americans compared to other communities. Therefore, you are at a higher risk of hypertension if you are African American.

Tobacco use: Cigarette smoking and tobacco chewing immediatelyraise blood pressure. Cigarettes contain harmful chemicals that cause damage to blood vessel walls. This causes them to narrow down, resulting in high blood pressure.

Physical inactivity: Leading a sedentary lifestyle with little or no physical activity will predispose you to high blood pressure. It is also likely to lead to weight problems and obesity. Those who are active tend to have a normal heart rate and normal blood pressure levels.

Being obese or overweight: Overweight and obese persons need more blood supply to their cells and tissues. This causes the heart to work harder to pump more blood which strains both the heart and the blood vessels. This tends to increase the risk of hypertension.

Excessive salt in diet: Consuming large quantities of salt in food can be dangerous. Sodium in salt or in a diet causes the body to retain fluid, and this can cause high blood pressure. It is also important to increase levels of potassium and vitamin D levels in any diet as a lack of these essential vitamins and minerals can elevate chances of suffering hypertension.

High-stress levels: It has been demonstrated that high-stress levels can cause a temporary rise in blood pressure. Unresolved stress and anxiety combined with tobacco use and excessive or binge eating can result in hypertension.

How to Prevent Against Hypertension and Stroke

It is important to take steps to prevent chronic conditions such as hypertension, stroke, and cardiovascular disease. Preventive steps are much better than cure or control. Here are some tips on how to prevent hypertension and stroke. The most important adjustments you can make include changing your lifestyle. If you can adapt to certain lifestyle habits and healthy eating, then you will improve your chances of preventing hypertension. The most important thing is to focus on the risk factors that can be changed.

1. Eat a balanced diet: It is important to eat a balanced diet with every meal. Healthy eating helps to keep your blood pressure under control. You need to consume plenty of fruits and vegetables and mostly those that are rich in potassium. Care should be taken to reduce the consumption of fat, excess calories, and sugars.

2. Reduce salt intake: It is very important to reduce salt intake and to cut back on sodium intake. Blood pressure increases relative to sodium intake. It is advisable to reduce or even cease consumption of processed and packaged foods which contain plenty of added salt.

3. Maintain a healthy body weight: One of the best ways of keeping hypertension at bay is to keep your weight down. Anyone who is overweight or obese should lose weight while anyone with normal weight should keep it that way. Regular workouts and healthy eating can help reduce body weight.

4. Lead an active lifestyle: One of the best ways of keeping hypertension at bay is to workout regularly. An active lifestyle where you engage in a regular physical activity is essential if you are to avoid hypertension. Regular exercises help you keep off the weight, burn calories, and regulate blood pressure. Doctors advise us to workout for at least 30 minutes at least 3 times per week.

5. Reduce alcohol intake: It is very important to limit alcohol intake as the years go by. High alcohol levels in the blood can result in hypertension. Generally, one standard drink per day should be sufficient.

6. Regular monitoring of blood pressure: Doctors advice that blood pressure be measured on a regular basis. The blood pressure can be measured at a doctor's office, a clinic, or even at home. This is very important because hypertension occurs without any visible signs or symptoms but can cause a lot of damage.

Alkaline Diet to Lower Blood Pressure

To lower blood pressure and for optimum health, it is advisable to consume alkaline foods. These foods help the body to maintain a slightly alkaline state. It is said that when the body is acidic, it is prone to disease, but in an alkaline state, no disease can thrive.

The standard American diet involves consumption of soft drinks, fast foods, grains, red meat, saturated fats, and artificial sweeteners, and so on. All these are highly acidic foods which are not good for your health.

Alkalizing foods helps to get rid of the acidity to reduce the risks of chronic conditions and diseases.

An acidic body lacks many essential minerals. It can result in inflammation and chronic conditions like arthritis and hypertension. The following alkaline foods are great for good health. They help lower blood pressure and maintain optimum health.

Vegetables

Kale, garlic, celery, mushrooms, onions, cabbages, carrots, broccoli, asparagus, mustard greens, cauliflower, Brussels sprouts, collard greens, wild greens, spirulina, peppers, peas, pumpkins, alfalfa, wheat grass, sea vegetables, etc.

Fruits

Pineapples, lemons, oranges, grapefruits, peaches, pears, watermelons, tropical fruits, avocados, dates, cherries, tangerines, limes, grapes, bananas, currants, tomatoes, apricots, apples, etc.

Proteins

Whey protein powder, nuts, chicken breasts, millet, tofu, eggs, cottage cheese, yogurt, sunflower seeds, almonds, squash seeds, sprouted seeds, pumpkin seeds, chestnut, etc.

Other alkaline foods

Ginseng tea, herbal tea, green tea, bee pollen, probiotic cultures, fresh fruit juice, organic milk, green juices, alkaline antioxidant water, and mineral water.

Other important tips for adding alkaline foods to a diet

It is important to add more fruits and vegetables to your diet. Having a large plate full of veggies is very important. Also, eating more vegetables in the night is absolutely important.

For snacks, a plate of cut-up veggies will do very well. Vegetables such as radishes, broccoli, celery, bell peppers, and cucumbers are perfect for snacks. Also, delicious fruit or vegetable juices are effective in alkalizing the entire body, and this helps lower blood pressure and improve health.

Some examples of juices that counter hypertension are listed below.

- Carrot, parsley, celery juice
- Whey powder and lime juice
- Pineapple and carrot juice with honey
- Carrot and grape juice
- Liquid Chlorophyll (you can get this at health food stores or online)
- Alfalfa, parsley, and pineapple juice

Chapter 5: Alkaline Diet and Cancer

For a long time now, there has been the belief that a diet that is low in acidic foods and high in alkaline foods can help fight or prevent cancer. It is known that cancer thrives in an acidic environment, but cannot survive in an alkaline one. Therefore, a diet that is high in alkaline foods, such as vegetables and fresh fruits, will raise the pH levels in the body, and this makes it difficult for cancer cells to thrive and survive.

Regulating Blood pH

Ordinarily, the lungs and kidneys regulate blood pH levels. However, oncologists such as Dr. Mitchell L Gaynor, M.D. of Gaynor Integrative Oncology, N.Y., agree that a low-acid diet helps fight and prevent cancer as it suppresses inflammation of the body. Ordinarily, blood pH levels range between 7.35 and 7.45 which is a little alkaline. While blood pH regulation is maintained by the lungs and kidneys, alkaline blood pH levels aid greatly in achieving this.

Early laboratory tests indicate that cancer cells actually thrive in acidic environments. However, some believe that cancer cells actually produce the acid in which they thrive through a process known as the Cori cycle.

Alkaline foods like nuts, root vegetables, fruits, fresh vegetables, and legumes are broken down during digestion into short-chain fatty acids. These short-chain fatty acids are rich in prebiotic nutrients which nourish gut bacteria. When these bacteria thrive, inflammation in the body decreases which is great in stifling cancer and hindering its growth.

Alkaline Diet and Cancer

Foods such as flour, saturated fats, and refined sugar tend to result in a highly acidic environment in the body. This acidic environment can easily result in inflammation, and it is in an inflamed body where cancer cells thrive.

According to research conducted in the UK, there is no evidence to support or disprove the fact that an alkaline diet can help cure cancer. This research can be found by **clicking on this link**. What is generally agreed upon is that an alkaline diet promotes good bacteria. Good bacteria help to reduce inflammation in the body and deny cancer the environment it needs to thrive.

Promoting the Alkaline Diet

It is important to eat healthy and generally lead a healthy lifestyle. This is generally the best way of avoiding chronic conditions such as cancer. Some individuals and companies promote their products, diet plans, and so on in an attempt to sell to vulnerable cancer patients.

Instead of buying expensive products such as alkaline water systems, it would be easier to transition into a healthy lifestyle. There are plenty of benefits of leading such a lifestyle.

Targeted Nutrition for Cancer

According to Dr. Sharon Gurm, a physician of oncology, it is better to follow dietary advice on how to eat to beat and survive cancer. This, she says, gives cancer patients the best chances of conquering cancer.

1. Follow a whole-foods based, low-glycemic diet that is rich in nutrients.
2. Stay hydrated and drink filtered water as often as possible.
3. Consume about 4 to 6 servings of vegetables everyday.
4. Minimize or avoid processed foods and alcohol as much as possible.

5. Conduct tests at a reputable lab to discover any food sensitivities.
6. There is no need to spend thousands of dollars on costly products.

If dietary supplements must be taken, then they should be from a trustworthy source and targeted to meet a specific need. There is a need to lead an active lifestyle. Research supports regular exercise for prevention and cure of cancer. In conclusion, it is obvious that beating cancer is a sum total of different activities and not just one intervention.

All around the world in countries like Japan, Canada, Germany, and the USA, oncologists are following an integrative cancer care protocol which makes use of both conventional and naturopathic therapies. There is mounting evidence that points to a better quality of life and survival rates when this dual approach is applied.

Chapter 6: Lowering Chronic Pain and Inflammation

Conditions such as chronic inflammation are usually as a result of the food we eat. Modern diets often consist of junk foods and processed foods. These tend to make our bodies very acidic. In fact, the more we consume these processed foods, the more acidic our bodies become.

Chronic Pain

Chronic pain is essentially pain that does not go away. We often feel pain when we hurt ourselves. This is common, but the pain eventually goes away. However, in cases where the pain is intense and lasts longer than 12 weeks, then it is known as chronic pain.

Inflammation can result in a condition such as fibromyalgia. The term fibromyalgia refers to a medical condition that is characterized by widespread, chronic muscle pain, sleep problems, painful tender points, and fatigue.

Problems Caused by Inflammation

When the body becomes too acidic, it results in a condition known as inflammation. Inflammation then causes other medical conditions such as allergies, asthma, arthritis, digestion problems, leaky gut, and food intolerance to occur. Medics now believe that inflammation plays a major role in conditions such as cancer, heart disease, obesity, and hypertension. Also, the more fat a person has, the more inflammation they have.

Modern Diets

A lot of diets that are popular today propose burning as many calories as those consumed. This is out of the belief that weight gain is a direct result of calories eaten. However, the body is more complicated than this. There are hormones, such as leptin, that help balance body weight. Chronic inflammation in the body also affects weight.

While many different factors can cause a system-wide inflammation, the biggest cause is, without a doubt, toxins within the body. These are toxins that result from the food we eat. A lot of the food we eat today is junk food that consists of toxins, highly processed sugars, and chemicals. Toxic overload results not just from unhealthy diets, but also from the pollution that is around us, and the water we drink, and plenty of harmful toxins in our environments.

While a lot of these toxins are eliminated via the skin, liver, kidneys, and so on, a lot of other toxins cannot be eliminated. These are instead stored as fat beneath the skin. Chronic inflammation is the major reason why people suffer from conditions such as obesity, heart disease, diabetes, and much more.

Solutions to Chronic Pain and Inflammation

The good news is that inflammation, chronic pain, and the resulting illnesses do not have to be a part of anyone's life. Such conditions can be managed, and most symptoms are likely to disappear if properly managed.

One of the most effective ways of getting rid of inflammation is turning to a healthy, alkaline diet. Eating foods that are alkaline in nature is extremely important. Also important are anti-inflammatory foods which largely target those suffering from chronic pain and conditions such as fibromyalgia. These foods provide a good defense against chronic inflammation and help to boost good health.

There are also detox diets available tailored specifically to address fibromyalgia. If fibromyalgia is addressed, then chronic pain and associated conditions like arthritis are likely to reduce in intensity with most pains and symptoms disappearing. The detox diets are tailored towards addressing chronic pain and are based only on foods that are alkaline in nature.

Meals that Treat Inflammation

Some of the best meals that we can have are obtained directly from the earth. The earth is full of nutrient-dense, healthy, natural, and alkaline foods. One of the best ways to tackle chronic pain with diet is to detoxify the liver. The liver should be detoxified with a healthy, natural diet that consists of natural, alkaline foods. Here are some of the most important alkaline foods that can help cleanse and detoxify your liver; thereby, getting rid of chronic pain, inflammation, and fibromyalgia.

1. Sarsaparilla: One of the best detox foods out there has to be sarsaparilla. It has been used as a diuretic for ages because it stimulates urination. A diuretic is an excellent choice for anyone who wants to detoxify the liver and get rid of toxins in their system. Sarsaparilla is also great for overall health.

2. Blue Vervain: Another great diuretic that is good for detox is blue vervain. It also helps to detoxify the liver by stimulating urination. When the liver is detoxified, harmful chemicals, fats, excess salt, and toxins are all removed from the body. This helps protect the liver and keep you healthy and pain-free eventually.

3. Coconut Oil: Coconut oil helps to prevent liver disease because it consists of medium-chain triglycerides. These can be converted into energy in the liver and help the liver with its workload. When the liver gets a break, and its workload is reduced, then it performs better and more efficiently.

4. Burdock tea: This tea is rather bitter, yet the ingredients that make it bitter can stimulate the production of important digestive juices such as bile in the stomach. These juices help to eliminate toxins from the body andkeep it healthy. As the liver eliminates toxins from the blood, it is aided by the ingredients found in burdock tea.

5. Prunes: Prunes are excellent for the liver. They help maintain healthy cholesterol and plasma levels.

6. Peaches: The peach is an excellent fruit that effectively detoxifies the liver. It cleanses the liver and helps eliminate the toxins that accumulate there. Peaches contain useful ingredients such as the hepatoprotectant. These are excellent for detoxifying and healing the liver. It is highly recommended for anyone seeking to cleanse their liver.

7. Goji Berries: This is a traditional fruit that has been used for ages to address liver conditions and to treat them. The goji berry is excellent at detoxifying the liver and eliminating toxins.

8. Bilberries: The bilberry is full of antioxidants and provides excellent protection to the liver against stress and damage. Scientific research indicates that the activity of bilberries reduces the levels of nitric oxide in the liver.

Chapter 7: How to Increase Absorption of Vitamins from Every Meal

We often endeavor to eat a healthy diet with every meal. Such a diet consists of all the important nutrients including essential vitamins, trace minerals, and much more. However, just because these important nutrients are in our meals does not mean that they get absorbed in the body. The body often misses out on the nutrition that it needs because these nutrients are not properly or adequately absorbed.

A recent study from the School of Medicine at Washington University indicates that bacteria found in the stomach play a major role in enabling the body to absorb nutrients. According to the study, healthy gut bacteria are necessary for proper nutrient absorption.

Also, some of the nutrients we take have poor bioavailability. This basically implies that the body finds it difficult to absorb essential nutrients. Fortunately, this does not have to be that way. You can easily increase nutrient absorption by proper food preparation.

How Exactly Does the Body Absorb Nutrients?

The body has digestive enzymes and bacteria that help to breakdown the food we eat. Food and everything else we eat is broken down into molecules which then enter the small intestines and then gets absorbed into the bloodstream. Once in the bloodstream, the nutrition then nourishes all the cells in the body.

However, absorption rates do vary. This variation ranges from 10% to almost 90% depending on certain factors. It is imperative that the body is enabled to absorb as much of the nutrients delivered as possible efficiently. If the body is inefficient at absorbing nutrients, malnutrition will set in. Other challenges will also follow. Fortunately, this is a challenge that can be overcome by following a couple of very simple steps. Here are some of the things you can do to improve nutrient absorption in the body.

1. Take Care of Your Gut

A lot of people may not know it, but the gut is home to over 100 trillion bacteria. Fortunately, these work in our favor and help to keep harmful bacteria at bay. It is a fact that over 80% of the human immune system cells are found in the intestines. Of these, gut microflora have a huge impact on your health and how you feel each day. Part of their function is to stimulate digestion and also absorption of nutrients.

However, these bacteria are under constant attack from processed foods, unhealthy fats, antibiotics, and lots of other toxic substances. Basically, a lot of what we consume each day puts gut bacteria under imminent threat, and this has a huge ramification on our health.

It is therefore advisable to take a regular probiotic supplement to help populate the good bacteria in the gut. When gut bacteria thrive, then proper nutritional absorption will take place.

2. Combine Different Food Types

Another great way of ensuring that your body receives all the nutrients it needs is to ensure that your diet consists of different types of food. A good diet should consist of healthy whole foods that grow in the ground. Combining these ensures your body is exposed to numerous essential nutrients, and that most will be absorbed.

3. Control Your Lifestyle

We lead fast and stressful lives, and this causes us to eat unhealthy meals including junk foods and all manner of processed foods. However, making a couple of adjustments can make a huge difference. For instance, we can start by consuming diets high in fiber and whole foods. We should also exercise regularly and avoid harmful substances and unhealthy food choices.

4. Introduce Healthy Fats into Your Diet

A lot of the important vitamins such as vitamins A, D, E, and K are all fat soluble. Therefore, if your body is to absorb all these essential vitamins, then you need to include healthy fats in your diet. Some of these fats include avocados, nuts, and even olive oil. Try to include them in your diet as often as you can. However, these should only be taken in moderation. Avoid saturated fats which come from dairy and meats. Plant-based fats are much better.

5. Prepare Meals Fast

Some nutrients such as B vitamins and C vitamins are water soluble. They tend to breakdown very easily especially when exposed to water and heat. Extended cooking methods such as baking and boiling should be avoided. Instead, fast cooking should be adopted such as steaming and baking.

6. Get the Sunshine Vitamin

Calcium is essential to the body, but for it to be absorbed, vitamin D is needed. In fact, lack of vitamin D can lead to calcium deficiency. It can be obtained from fatty fish like salmon and even from fortified milk. Exposure to sunlight also helps. Scientists recommended exposure to sunlight about 3 to 4 times a week without any suntan lotion.

7. Boost Digestive Enzymes

There are common digestive enzymes found in the gut. These include lactase, amylase, and protease. While they are produced in the small intestine, they can also be obtained in raw, unprocessed foods such as papayas and pineapples.

8. Add Aloe Vera to Your Diet

Aloe vera greatly helps with the absorption of vitamins in the body. Research studies from the UC Davis Medical Center have shown that aloe vera greatly enhances the absorption of vitamin C and vitamin B12. More about this study by UC Davies can be found here.

Chapter 8: Using the Alkaline Diet for Effective, Long-Term Weight Loss

The Alkaline Diet

It has been established that the alkaline diet, also known as the ash diet or alkaline acid diet, helps prevent problems such as cancer and arthritis. It also helps to reduce weight.

The theory behind this approach is that certain foods, such as refined sugars and junk food, cause the body to produce acid which is bad for your health and causes harmful substances to be converted to fat. However, an alkaline diet consists of the right nutrients and elements and therefore helps the body to lose weight.

Alkaline Body State

The alkaline diet needs the body to be in alkaline or at least a neutral state for it to perform optimally. Therefore, reducing the intake of foods that cause an increase in the amount of acid in the body should be reduced. Instead, you should follow a diet that causes the body and blood to be alkaline. Only natural, healthy, unprocessed foods cause the body to be alkaline. They are rich in nutrients, vitamins, and minerals.

Foods that You Can Eat

There are certain foods that you are allowed to eat. These include most fruits and most vegetables. For instance, seeds, nuts, tofu, and soybeans are all great and good for an alkaline diet. You are really allowed to consume anything that grows directly from the ground. These foods contain essential nutrients that the body requires, and so they will be absorbed by the body.

Alkaline Herbs

Generally, all herbs are considered alkaline. One of the most powerful herbs and superfoods is garlic. It always ranks at the top of most food lists and is an alkaline herb. It helps regulate pH, lower blood pressure and is great for weight loss. Other herbs that are recommended for weight loss include cayenne pepper, bell peppers, parsley, and dill weed.

Foods You Are Not Allowed to Eat

There are certain foods that are not part of an alkaline diet. For instance, dairy products are not good for the body because they cause acidity. It is far better to consume soy milk and other products instead.

Other foods that are forbidden include junk foods, processed foods, red meat, convenience foods, packaged snacks, eggs, and most grains. The problem with these foods is that they are not natural, but contain a lot of hazardous chemicals, toxins, and very little nutrition. Even alcohol is not allowed. When consumed, the toxins and other substances are converted into fat and stored in the body usually in the arteries and veins. The fat is also stored around the waist and stomach area.

When you switch to an alkaline diet, you will lose weight because the good, natural food that you consume is absorbed by the body, and any waste is eliminated. This will ensure that very little waste is converted into fat and stored in the body. Also, the body will be able to breakdown the fat and eliminate it from the body.

On the other hand, consumption of processed foods and unhealthy options such as dairy and grains will result in increased weight and stored fat. Therefore, adopting an alkaline diet is advisable for weight loss. You should eat more natural products and reduce your intake of refined sugars and processed foods for a healthy body and weight loss.

Spices for Weight Loss

1. Green tea: Green tea helps with weight loss because it contains plenty of antioxidants. It also speeds up metabolism. It is recommended to drink 4 to 5 cups of green tea throughout the day to reduce weight.

2. Ginseng: This herb is also recommended for weight loss. It also helps regulate diabetes. As a ground herb, ginseng can be added to food or tea. Simply add one teaspoon to any meal. As a beverage, ginseng should be boiled in water for about 45 minutes. One ginseng root can be boiled then honey, and cinnamon added.

3. Turmeric: This is a bright yellow spice that is excellent for burning fat and also detoxifying the liver. This is according to research undertaken at Tufts University. The active ingredient in turmeric is known as curcumin, and it hastens metabolism. Turmeric can be chopped up or ground and added to soup or stew until the taste is palatable enough. It can also be taken as a drink. Simply add 2 knobs of turmeric in hot water then add some lemon and honey and mix to taste.

4. Hibiscus: This is a beautiful flower that is packed rich with minerals, flavonoids, and nutrients. Hibiscus breaks down the fats and carbohydrates, and they are then flushed out of the body. For weight loss, you will need 2 dried hibiscus leaves, 2 cups of water, and 1 tablespoon of honey for sweetening. Heat the water and add the hibiscus leaves. Boil the leaves, then strain and pour into a cup.

Chapter 9: 7-Day Alkaline Diet Eating Plan

An alkaline diet has many benefits as has already been established. Not only does it help improve overall health, but also aids in weight loss and reduces inflammation. An alkaline body provides protection against numerous conditions such as hypertension, arthritis, heart disease, and many more.

An appropriate alkaline diet should consist of foods that help to balance the body's pH levels. Here is a 7-day diet plan that consists of healthy alkaline foods. This particular eating plan has been developed by two experts. One is Natasha Corrett, an organic chef, and the other is nutritional therapist Nicky Edgson. These experts are of the opinion that an optimum body pH can be achieved via a 20% acidic and an 80% alkaline diet.

Regulations of this Diet

Within this 7-day period, the only foods to be consumed are beans, peas, tofu, legumes, fruits, nuts, vegetables, seeds, and healthy fats. The healthy fats include olive oil, coconut oil, and flaxseed.

One more thing to note, there are no requirements regarding meal timing, you can simply eat when you are hungry.

Day 1

Breakfast: Strawberry and chia seed quinoa

Snack: One orange fruit

Lunch: A fruit and a half bowl of vegetable salad

Snack: A half cup of dried fruits and roasted nuts

Dinner

2 pieces of Roasted chicken

1 ½ roasted sweet potatoes,

Veggie salad with olive oil

Veggie Salad Ingredients:

½ sliced cucumber

1 cubed avocado

1 pomegranate

½ cup shelled and chopped pistachios

Chia Seed and Strawberry Quinoa

6 tablespoons of chia seeds

4 sliced strawberries and 1/3 cup quartered

strawberries

1.5 cups of cooked quinoa

2 cups of coconut milk

2 pitted dates

3 tablespoons of unsweetened coconut flakes and chopped almonds

Preparation

Prepare the quinoa a day earlier. Prepare the puree by blending the coconut milk with the dates. Pour the puree in a jar then add chia seeds. Stir the mixture then cover and refrigerate overnight. During breakfast, pour the chia seeds and quinoa in a bowl. You can add any toppings you like.

Day 2

Breakfast: blueberry, raspberry, and strawberry smoothie

Snack: 3 slices of pineapple

Lunch: 4 ounces Noodles and sesame dressing

Snack: A small plate of dried apricot fruit

Dinner: 4 ounces of roasted salmon, ½ baked sweet potato,

¼ pound of green vegetables

Sesame Dressing

¼ cup of distilled water

2 large garlic cloves

1 tablespoon of minced ginger

¼ cup natural peanut butter

½ cup of coconut oil

3 tablespoons of sesame oil

½ lime

½ cup of soy sauce

Smoothie ingredients

2 cups of almond milk

2 ½ cups of fresh spinach

1 tablespoon chia seeds

1 frozen banana

1 cup of mixed berries and strawberries

Day 3

Breakfast: Apple parfait

Snack: A single mango fruit

Lunch: White bean stew and avocado wraps

Snack: A cup of toasted pumpkin seeds

Dinner: 3 to 4 ounces of roasted chicken, 1 plate
cucumber salad, roasted,

1 ½ pounds of Brussels sprout with 1 tablespoon of
olive oil and ½ tablespoon apple cider vinegar

Vegan apple parfait ingredients

1 cup of rolled uncooked oats

½ cup of unsweetened coconut milk

½ tablespoon vanilla extract

1 tablespoon hemp seeds

1 cup chopped apples

Avocado wrap ingredients

1 collard leaf bunch

½ diced red onion

Sea salt and pepper to taste

1 sliced and chopped tomato

Handful of spinach leaves

½ an avocado fruit

Day 4

Breakfast: Almond and apple butter oats

Snack: 1 ripe banana

Lunch: Avocado cumin and lemon dressing

Snack: One cup of almonds

Dinner: Zucchini noodles and kale pesto

Almond and apple butter oats ingredients

2.5 cups of oats

1 cup coconut milk

¼ cup raw almond butter

1.5 cups of grated green apple

A dash of cinnamon

Avocado cumin ingredients

1 avocado

2 freshly squeezed limes

A dash of black pepper

1 cup of water

1 ½ teaspoons of cumin powder

½ teaspoon sea salt

½ tablespoon of virgin olive oil

½ freshly squeezed lemon

Salad ingredients

1 zucchini

1/3 cup of soaked and drained kelp noodles

4 cups of chopped kale

2 ½ tablespoons hemp seeds

½ cup of chopped broccoli

Day 5

Breakfast: A power smoothie

Snack: 1 mango

Lunch: Quinoa burrito bowl

Snack: One cup of dates

Dinner: Almond risotto and wild rice with mushrooms

Power smoothie ingredients

2 ½ cups of spinach

2 tablespoons almond butter

1 frozen banana

1 ½ tablespoons of coconut oil

½ tablespoon cinnamon

2 cups of almond milk

1 cup of mixed berries

Mix all the ingredients in a blender thoroughly and then pour into a cup

Quinoa burrito bowl

4 minced garlic cloves

2 cans of black beans

1 tablespoon cumin seeds

2 freshly squeezed limes

2 sliced avocados

1 cup of quinoa

3 large green onions, sliced

Handful of chopped cilantro

Cook the quinoa then heat beans in a skillet over low heat. Now add the onions, garlic, and cumin and lime juice then cook for 15 minutes. Now add the avocado and fresh cilantro.

Day 6

Breakfast: Quinoa porridge

Snack: 3 to 4 cantaloupe slices

Lunch: Mexican quinoa salad

Snack: 1 cup of mixed nuts and dried coconut

Dinner: 1 bowl pumpkin soup

Mexican quinoa salad ingredients

14 ounces or 1 can of corn

½ cup of chopped cilantro

1 chopped red bell pepper

1 can or 14 ounces of pinto beans

15 ounces or 1 can of kidney beans

2 ½ cups of cooked quinoa

1 chopped red onion

1 cup of cooked brown rice

Add all ingredients in a glass bowl and mix thoroughly.

Prepare a dressing and pour it on top

Quinoa porridge ingredients

1 can or 15 ounces of coconut milk

½ tablespoon hemp seeds

½ tablespoon chia seeds

1 teaspoon cinnamon

¾ cup of rinsed quinoa

Mix all ingredients in a small saucepan except the hemp seed. Let the mixture simmer for about 15 to 18 minutes then add the hemp seed.

Pumpkin Soup

2 sugar pumpkins

1 cup of coconut milk

2 tablespoons of honey

3 cups of veggie broth

Day 7

Breakfast: Fresh chia seed pudding

Snack: ½ a small cup of blueberries

Lunch: Fermented tofu and miso soup

Snack: Small cup of macadamia nuts

Dinner: 4 ounces of salmon and roasted vegetables

Chia seed pudding ingredients

1 cup of coconut milk

5 tablespoons chia seeds

½ a cup of chopped nuts (cashew, hazelnuts, or almonds)

¼ cup of vanilla extract

½ a teaspoon of cinnamon

1 tablespoon of shredded and unsweetened coconut flakes

Take a jar and mix the chia seeds with the milk. Now add the chopped nuts, vanilla, and cinnamon. Stir the mix and then refrigerate overnight. Shake it in the morning and add nuts, fresh fruits, and coconut shreds.

Roasted vegetable ingredients

I pounds of cut and peeled parsnips,

2 tablespoons of fresh chopped rosemary

1 ½ pounds of chopped, unpeeled potatoes, chopped into pieces

2 chopped leeks

1 pound of chopped and peeled celery root

¾ pounds of carrots, peeled and chopped up

9 peeled, garlic cloves

2 tablespoons of extra virgin olive oil

Preheat oven to 400 degrees F. Mix ingredients minus the garlic in a bowl then bake in the oven for 30 minutes. Reverse positions, add the garlic and bake for another half hour.

Summer Green Smoothie Bowl

Ingredients

1 banana

2 cups of almond milk

1 small mango cut into chunks

2 tablespoons of hulled hemp seeds

Half-medium sliced cucumber

1 tablespoon of moringa powder

A handful of kale or spinach

1 half cup of soaked almonds

Preparation

Put all the different ingredients in a blender then blend the mixture until it becomes creamy and smooth. Now add some water or milk and blend some more. Pour the final blend into a bowl and top it up with granola, coconut, and pumpkin seeds.

Acai Berry Smoothie Bowl

Ingredients

1 banana, frozen or fresh

2 teaspoons of maca powder

3 tablespoons of acai powder

Cacao

1 tablespoon of organic maple syrup

2 tablespoons of cashews or almonds

1 cup of mixed berries or blueberries

Toppings

¼ teaspoon chia seeds

Handful of dried coconut

½ cup of yogurt

Handful of almonds

Method

Blend the acai, berries, maca, banana, nuts, and cacao together. Add sweetener and milk and continue to blend until smooth. Add more milk if necessary. Now add the toppings such as chia seeds, coconut yogurt, and almond seeds.

Imitation Starbucks Pumpkin Latte, Limited Ingredients

Ingredients

1 teaspoon of vanilla syrup

½ cup of whipped cream

1 cup of almond milk

1 cup of coffee or espresso

Pumpkin spice with ginger, nutmeg, or cinnamon to garnish

1 tablespoon of pumpkin spice syrup

Preparation method

Add the pumpkin spice syrup, milk, and vanilla syrup in a Mason jar.

Seal the jar then shake until the milk doubles in volume and becomes frothy.

Unseal the jar and place in a microwave oven for 2 minutes until the milk is steamed. Pour the milk into the coffee or espresso then top it up with pumpkin spice seasoning or whipped cream.

Chapter 10: Alkaline Juice Recipes

1. Lemon Ginger Alkaline Juice

Ingredients

1 teaspoon of apple cider vinegar

1-inch long piece of ginger

Preparation Method

Add the lemon and ginger in a blender. Juice the mixture and add some water if necessary. Now add the apple cider vinegar and mix some more. The juice is ready to serve.

2. Sweet Green Alkaline Juice

Ingredients

A handful of fresh mint

A bunch of Swiss chard

1 cucumber

A tablespoon of chia seeds

1 pear

Method

Chop the Swiss chard and roll up the leaves. No need to peel the pear, but it should be chopped as well. Add the Swiss chard, cucumber, mint, and pear into the juicer. Mix these for 2 minutes then add the pear.

3. Green Zinger Alkaline Juice

Ingredients

1 lemon

2 pears

2 cucumbers

A handful of string beans

2-inch piece of ginger

2 tablespoons of chia seeds

Method

Chop up the ingredients, pour them into a blender, and blend for 2 to 3 minutes. Remove from blender, and pour into a bowl. Add the chia seeds at this stage, and then use a cappuccino whisk to mix the chia seeds with the juice. This will enable the seeds to expand and soften then spread throughout the juice mixture.

4. PH Booster Green Juice

Ingredients

One half-peeled lemon

3 to 4 celery stalks

2 cucumbers

Method

Simply cut the ingredients into sized chunks then throw them into the blender
Blend for 2 to 3 minutes then pour into a glass and enjoy.

Chapter 11: How to Keep Food Costs Down

Food prices have been going up over the years while incomes have either remained stagnant or been reduced. This necessitates the need to keep food costs down. Here are a couple of ways of bringing down food costs to manageable levels.

1. Dine in

Dining out regularly is quite expensive. Any meals you consume at a restaurant can be prepared at home at a fraction of the cost. There is no need to go out for junk food because they are harmful to your health though they are cheap.

2. Stock up

It is important to buy in bulk to realize some savings. Whenever you are out shopping, be sure to check the prices. If bulk items are available, they are very likely to be cheaper than standard items.

3. Sign up for Reward Schemes

Most stores offer reward cards and other benefits. Learn to take advantage of these as they can save you money in the long run.

4. Lookout for Discounts

Most stores offer discounted prices on certain items pretty regularly. It is important to be a smart shopper and find items that, for instance, are very close to their sell-by dates. Such items are often available at a discount.

5. Pay in Cash

You should ensure you pay cash for all your groceries. When credit cards are used, they may cost you more if you do not pay them off in full at the end of the month. Rather than pay the extra costs, it is much easier to pay in cash.

6. Use Coupons

Coupons offer an excellent method of saving money on your grocery shopping. Find coupons offered by your store, and use them the next time you go grocery shopping.

7. Buy in Season

This is an important but grossly overlooked one. Fruit and vegetables can often to be up to 50% cheaper if you buy them while in season. So take a look online for the seasons for various foods, and when you go to the store - buy more of the ones which are in season vs. the more expensive out of season foods

Chapter 12: Is Alkaline Water Worthy or Just a Fad?

What is Alkaline Water?

Lately - we've been seeing a surge in the popularity of certain waters marketed as "alkaline water". These are bottles of water sold at a significant markup as opposed to regular bottled water. Now - as an author I feel it necessary to deeply investigate Alkaline water is the opposite of acidic water.

Alkaline water is the opposite of acidic water. This is water with a pH level above 7. Ordinary or plain water is supposed to have a neutral pH or 7. There have been claims that alkaline water is healthy and beneficial to the body. This has made alkaline water very popular around the world.

The pH of rainwater is slightly lower than 7 because of absorbed carbon dioxide. Carbon dioxide increases the acidity of water. According to the *Medical News Today* journal, alkaline water has some benefits. This means it is not just a fad. These facts have been checked and approved by their medical review team led by Natalie Butler, RD, LD.

Effects of Alkaline Water on the Body

1. According to research, calcium and bicarbonate-rich alkali mineral water do not have a huge effect on osteoporosis. Scientists believe more research is needed in this instance.

2. When it comes to cancer, there were studies conducted to check whether alkaline water has any effect on cancer. Based on the research, alkaline water did not necessarily improve cancer, but an alkaline diet enhanced the action of chemotherapy drugs.

3. Alkaline water was found to stop enzymes that cause acid reflux. This is according to a study published in the *Annals of Otology, Rhinology, and Laryngology*. Alkaline water also appeared to minimize acidity in the stomach to reasonable levels.

4. Alkaline water helps to reduce blood pressure and to lower blood sugar levels. This conclusion is based on a study by scientists in Shanghai who studied patients between 3 and 6 months. This study can be found in the 2001 issue of the *Shanghai Journal of Preventive Medicine*. Therefore, drinking alkaline water can help reduce high blood pressure, high blood lipids, and high blood sugar.

Conclusion

And there we have it, hopefully this book has cleared up any questions you had about the life changing positive effects of the alkaline diet. From weight loss, to improving your overall wellbeing and reducing chronic pain - this diet is changing thousands of people's lives around the world, and I hope you become one of them.

Remember this, some of these changes can result in positive effects in as little as one week, others may take more time for you to see - but rest assured, by eating the right foods you will get the right results.

Diet is only one part of a healthy lifestyle, exercise is equally as important - not just for your physical but also your mental health. I recommend a minimum of 45 minutes of moderate exercise 4 times a week. If you're not in a position to do this then even small changes like taking the stairs instead of the elevator at work (providing you don't work on the 54th floor!) can make a big difference.

Finally - I hope you've enjoyed this book and if you have - I'd appreciate it if you left a review on Amazon.

Thanks,

Jason Michaels

Other Books by Jason Michaels

Anti-Inflammatory Diet: How You Can Lose Up to 25lbs and Reduce Belly Fat Before Swimsuit Season

www.ingramcontent.com/pod-product-compliance
Lightning Source LLC
Chambersburg PA
CBHW050750030426
42336CB00012B/1741